2024 ULTIMATE WEIGHT POINT COOKBOOK

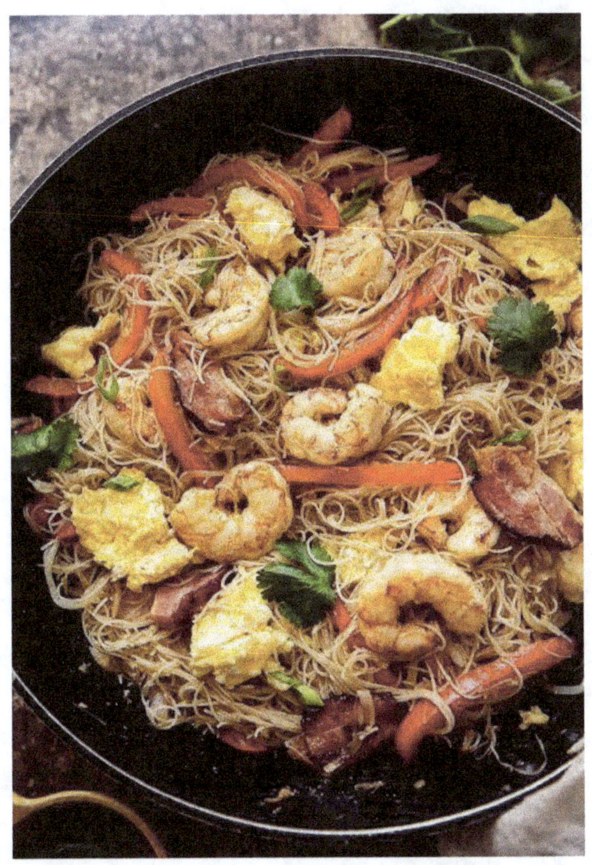

Healthy Potassium Foods, Low-Calorie Recipes, and Nutritional Guidance - Illustrated for Beginners & Pros

Publisher's Note

Table of contents

Dedication

Dear Beloved Readers,

This cookbook is a heartfelt dedication to each of you embarking on a beautiful journey toward better health and happiness. Your decision to prioritize your well-being is a testament to your strength and commitment to self-love.

May these pages unfold a tapestry of culinary joy, guiding you through delicious recipes crafted with care. Each dish is not just a meal; it's a celebration of your journey—one that intertwines flavor, nutrition, and the pursuit of your healthiest, happiest self.

Here's to savoring the joy of nourishing your body and relishing every moment of your transformative adventure.

With warmth and encouragement,

Oamal Christian.

USER'S GUIDE

Welcome to a transformative experience with the "2024 Ultimate Weight Point Cookbook." To ensure your journey is not only enjoyable but highly effective in managing your weight and enhancing your health, consider these comprehensive tips:

1. Embrace Variety for Nutritional Riches:

- Explore the diverse array of recipes within the cookbook to ensure you benefit from a broad spectrum of nutrients crucial for overall well-being. Embracing variety not only enhances your palate but also contributes to a balanced, nourishing diet.

2. Plan Your Culinary Week:

- Take a proactive approach by planning your weekly meals using the cookbook. This not only streamlines your grocery shopping but also sets the stage for a week of mindful, health-conscious eating.

3. Master Portion Control:

- While our recipes are crafted to be both flavorful and satisfying, understanding portion control is key. Be mindful of serving sizes to align your meals with your specific dietary requirements and weight management goals.

4. Stay Hydrated for Optimal Health:

   - Water is your ally in weight management. Ensure you stay well-hydrated throughout the day to support your metabolism, aid digestion, and reduce the likelihood of confusing thirst with hunger.

5. Listen to Your Body's Signals:

   - Cultivate a deeper connection with your body by paying attention to hunger and fullness cues. Eating when genuinely hungry and stopping when satisfied fosters a healthier relationship with food.

6. Integrate Regular Exercise:

   - Complement your culinary adventures with regular physical activity. Whether it's a brisk walk, yoga session, or hitting the gym, incorporating exercise enhances the positive impact of your weight management journey.

7. Seek Support in Community:

   - Share your experiences with friends or family, creating a supportive community. Engaging with others can provide motivation, opportunities for recipe swaps, and a shared commitment to healthier living.

8. Personalize Recipes to Suit You:

   - Feel empowered to customize recipes based on your taste preferences and dietary needs. Cooking is a flexible and enjoyable experience that should seamlessly align with your lifestyle.

9. Track Your Culinary Progress:

   - Keep a journal to document your culinary triumphs, noting how certain recipes make you feel, and tracking any positive changes in your weight and overall well-being. Celebrate each step forward in your journey.

10. Consistency is the Foundation:

   - Sustainable results arise from consistent efforts. While savoring the culinary delights of our cookbook, remember that lasting success is built upon a foundation of healthy habits cultivated over time.

As you immerse yourself in the "2024 Ultimate Weight Point Cookbook," recognize it not merely as a recipe book but as a guiding companion on your transformative path to better health and vitality. Here's to a healthier, more vibrant you!

INTRODUCTION

Welcome to the "2024 Ultimate Weight Point Cookbook," where we go on a transforming culinary journey together. In the pages that follow, you'll find not just a collection of recipes but a full guide to altering your relationship with food, fostering weight loss, and embracing a healthy lifestyle.

What Awaits You:

1. Healthy Potassium Foods: - Delve into a world of cuisine precisely designed around potassium-rich ingredients. These important nutrients contribute not just to a balanced diet but also play a crucial role in overall health. From the succulence of salmon to the freshness of leafy greens, our meals are a celebration of good, nourishing ingredients.

2. Low-Calorie Delights: - Bid farewell to the assumption that low-calorie equals boring and uninspiring. Our cookbook defies this concept by delivering a varied assortment of foods that are both tempting to the taste buds and friendly to your waistline. From soul-warming chilies to delectable grilled proteins, each recipe is a tribute to the delight of conscious, savoury dining.

3. Nutritional Guidance: - Knowledge is power, especially when it comes to making informed choices about what goes into your body. In this cookbook, we provide expert dietary guidance. Understand the advantages of each component, grasp the entire nutritional profile of your meals, and empower yourself to make health-conscious decisions that coincide with your wellness goals.

4. Illustrated for Beginners & Pros: - Visualize your culinary wonders before they even hit the dish. Our cookbook is not just a compilation of recipes; it's an entire experience. Vibrant visuals accompany each meal, guaranteeing that whether you're a kitchen newbie or an expert chef, you can confidently bring these delicious delights to life.

Why This Cookbook?

In a society saturated with quick cures and restrictive diets, we hold firm in our view that permanent weight management begins with a love for great, nourishing food. Our recipes are a testament to this concept, reaching the perfect mix between flavor, nutrition, and simplicity. Whether you're commencing on your health journey or seeking fresh, interesting recipes to boost your cooking talents, this cookbook is your go-to reference.

So, take your apron, dive into these pages, and appreciate the thrill of nourishing your body with every exquisite meal. Welcome to a healthier, more vibrant self. The "2024 Ultimate Weight Point Cookbook" is more than a cookbook; it's a blueprint to a lifestyle that embraces the beauty of balanced, tasty food.

Blueberry Muffins

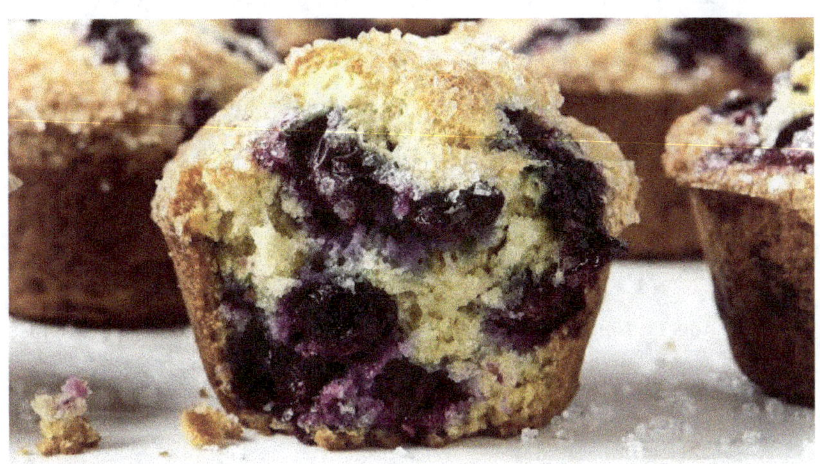

Ingredients:

- 1 cup all-purpose flour

- 1 cup whole wheat flour

- 1/4 cup sugar (or a sugar substitute like erythritol)

- 1 1/2 teaspoons baking powder

- 1/2 teaspoon baking soda

- 1/4 teaspoon salt

- 1 cup nonfat Greek yogurt - 2 large eggs

- 1/4 cup unsweetened applesauce

- 1 teaspoon vanilla extract

- 1 1/2 cups fresh or frozen blueberries

Instructions:

1. Preheat the oven to 350°F (175°C) and line a muffin tin with paper liners.

2. In a large bowl, whisk together the flours, sugar, baking powder, baking soda, and salt.

3. In another bowl, mix the Greek yogurt, eggs, applesauce, and vanilla extract until well combined.

4. Add the wet ingredients to the dry ingredients and stir until just combined.

5. Gently fold in the blueberries.

6. Spoon the batter into the muffin cups, filling each about 2/3 full.

7. Bake for 18-20 minutes or until a toothpick inserted into the center comes out clean.

8. Allow the muffins to cool in the tin for 5 minutes before transferring to a wire rack.

Notes:

- Opt for a sugar substitute to reduce the overall sugar content.

- Ensure the yogurt is non-fat.

Peanut Butter Pie

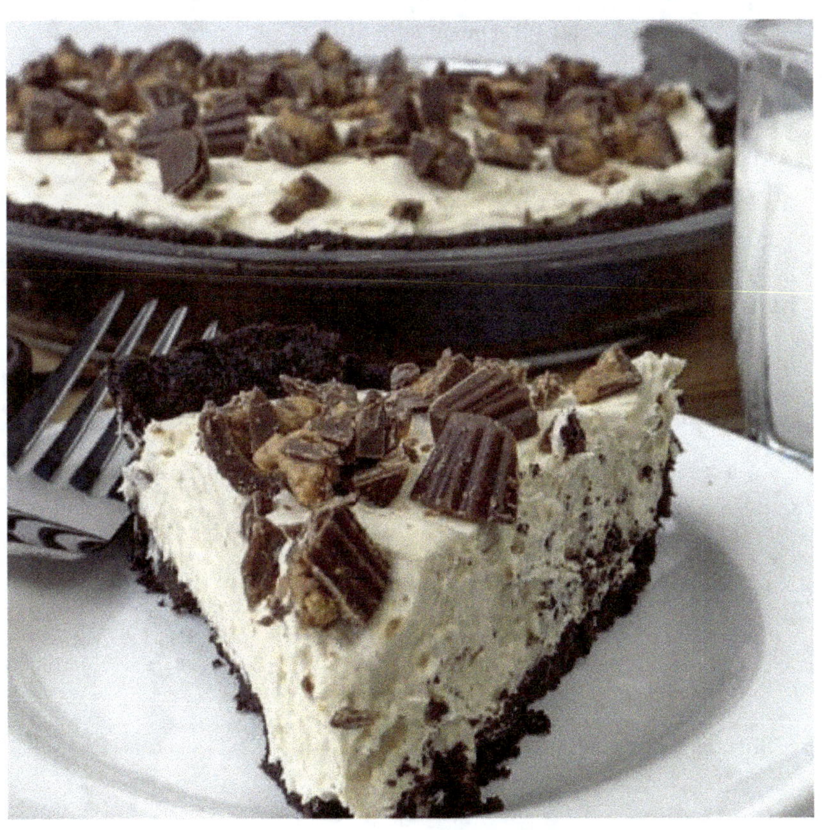

Ingredients:

- 1 1/2 cups crushed graham cracker crumbs (consider reduced-fat or sugar-free)

- 2 tablespoons melted butter (use a reduced-fat option)

- 1 cup powdered peanut butter (reconstituted with water to your desired consistency)

- 1 cup powdered sugar (or a sugar substitute)

- 8 oz reduced-fat cream cheese, softened

- 1 teaspoon vanilla extract

- 1 1/2 cups fat-free whipped topping

Instructions:

1. In a bowl, combine the graham cracker crumbs and melted butter. Press the mixture into the bottom of a pie dish to form the crust.

2. In a large bowl, beat together the powdered peanut butter, powdered sugar, cream cheese, and vanilla extract until smooth.

3. Fold in the whipped topping until well combined.

4. Spoon the peanut butter mixture into the crust and spread it evenly.

5. Refrigerate for at least 4 hours or until set.

6. Slice and serve chilled.

Notes:

- Use reduced-fat or sugar-free graham crackers for the crust.

- Opt for powdered peanut butter to reduce the fat content.

- Consider a sugar substitute to lower the sugar content.

3. Chicken Lettuce Wraps

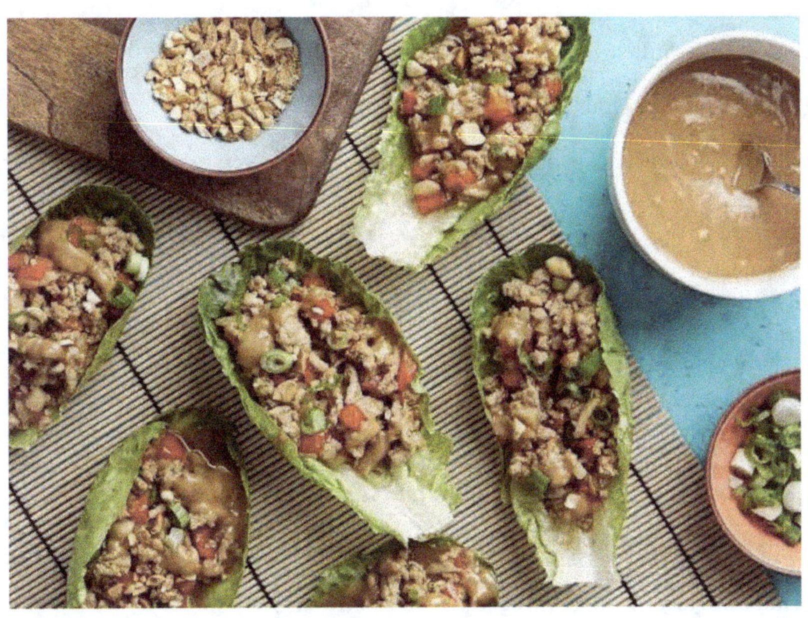

Ingredients:

- 1 lb ground chicken

- 1 tbsp olive oil - 1 onion, diced

- 2 cloves garlic, minced

- 1/4 cup soy sauce

- 2 tbsp hoisin sauce

- 1 tbsp rice vinegar

- 1 tsp ginger, grated

- 1 cup water chestnuts, chopped

- 1/4 cup green onions, sliced - 1 head iceberg lettuce

Instructions:

1. Cook ground chicken in olive oil.

2. Add onion, garlic, soy sauce, hoisin sauce, rice vinegar, and ginger. Cook until onions are soft.

3. Stir in water chestnuts and green onions.

4. Spoon mixture into lettuce leaves.

Tips:

Use lean ground chicken for a healthier option.

Opt for low-sodium soy sauce to reduce sodium intake.

Add a variety of colorful vegetables for extra nutrients.

Nutritional Information (per serving):

Calories: 250

Protein: 20g

Carbohydrates: 12g

Fat: 14g

Fiber: 3g

4. Skinny Cobb Salad

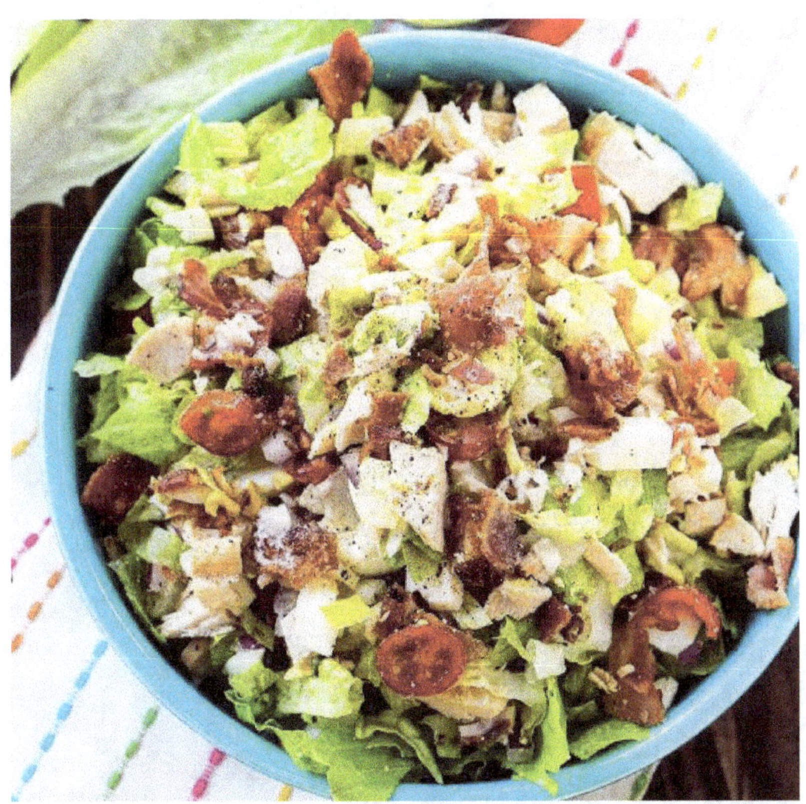

Ingredients:

- 2 cups mixed salad greens

- 1 cup grilled chicken, diced

- 1/2 cup cherry tomatoes, halved

- 1/4 cup cucumber, sliced

- 2 hard-boiled eggs, sliced

- 2 slices turkey bacon, crumbled

- 1/4 cup blue cheese, crumbled

- 2 tbsp balsamic vinaigrette

Instructions:

1. Arrange salad greens on a plate.

2. Top with grilled chicken, cherry tomatoes, cucumber, hard-boiled eggs, turkey bacon, and blue cheese.

3. Drizzle with balsamic vinaigrette.

Tips:

Choose grilled chicken breast for a lean protein source.

Use a mix of dark leafy greens for added vitamins and minerals.

Control portion sizes of bacon and cheese for a balanced salad.

Nutritional Information (per serving):

Calories: 350

Protein: 25g

Carbohydrates: 15g

Fat: 20g

Fiber: 5g

5. Tortilla Pinwheels

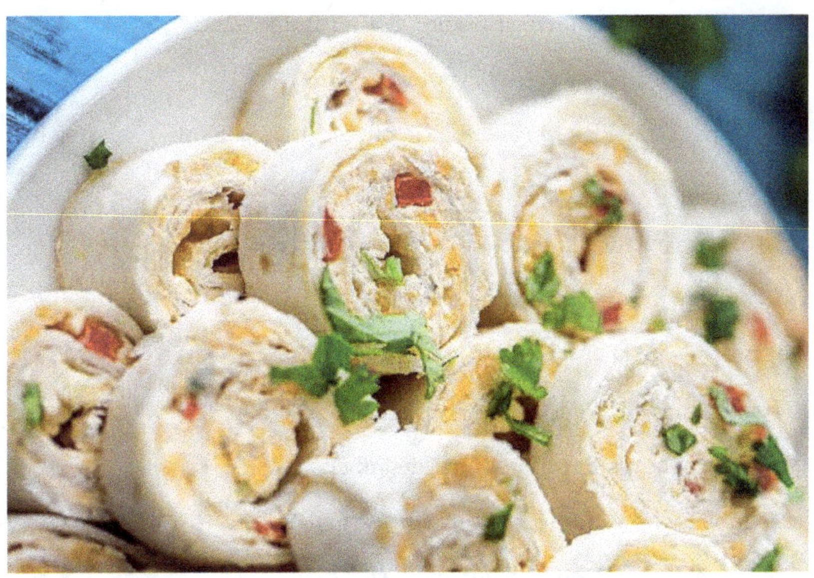

Ingredients:

- 8 oz cream cheese, softened

- 1 cup salsa

- 1 cup shredded cheddar cheese

- 1/2 cup black olives, sliced

- 1/4 cup green onions, chopped

- 1/4 cup red bell pepper, diced

- 6 large tortillas

Instructions:

1. In a bowl, mix cream cheese and salsa until smooth.

2. Spread the mixture evenly over tortillas.

3. Sprinkle cheddar cheese, black olives, green onions, and red bell pepper.

4. Roll up each tortilla tightly and refrigerate for an hour.

5. Slice into pinwheels before serving.

Tips:

Opt for whole-grain tortillas for added fiber.

Customize with your favorite salsa for extra flavor.

Prepare ahead for a convenient and healthy snack.

Nutritional Information (per serving):

Calories: 180

Protein: 8g

Carbohydrates: 15g

Fat: 10g

Fiber: 2g

6. Stuffed Pepper Soup

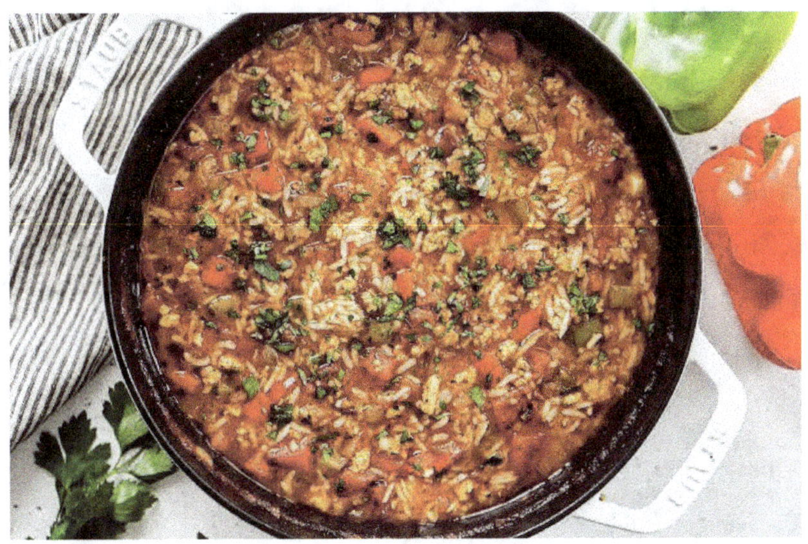

Ingredients:

- 1 lb ground turkey

- 1 onion, diced

- 2 bell peppers, diced

- 2 cloves garlic, minced

- 1 can (14 oz) diced tomatoes

- 1 can (14 oz) tomato sauce

- 4 cups chicken broth

- 1 cup brown rice, cooked

- 1 tsp Italian seasoning

- Salt and pepper to taste

Instructions:

1. In a pot, cook ground turkey until browned.

2. Add onion, bell peppers, and garlic. Cook until vegetables are tender.

3. Stir in diced tomatoes, tomato sauce, chicken broth, cooked rice, and Italian seasoning.

4. Simmer for 15-20 minutes. Season with salt and pepper.

Tips:

Use lean ground turkey to reduce saturated fat.

Increase vegetable variety for added vitamins.

Consider adding quinoa or brown rice for extra fiber.

Nutritional Information (per serving):

Calories: 220

Protein: 18g

Carbohydrates: 25g

Fat: 7g

Fiber: 6g

7. Cabbage Soup

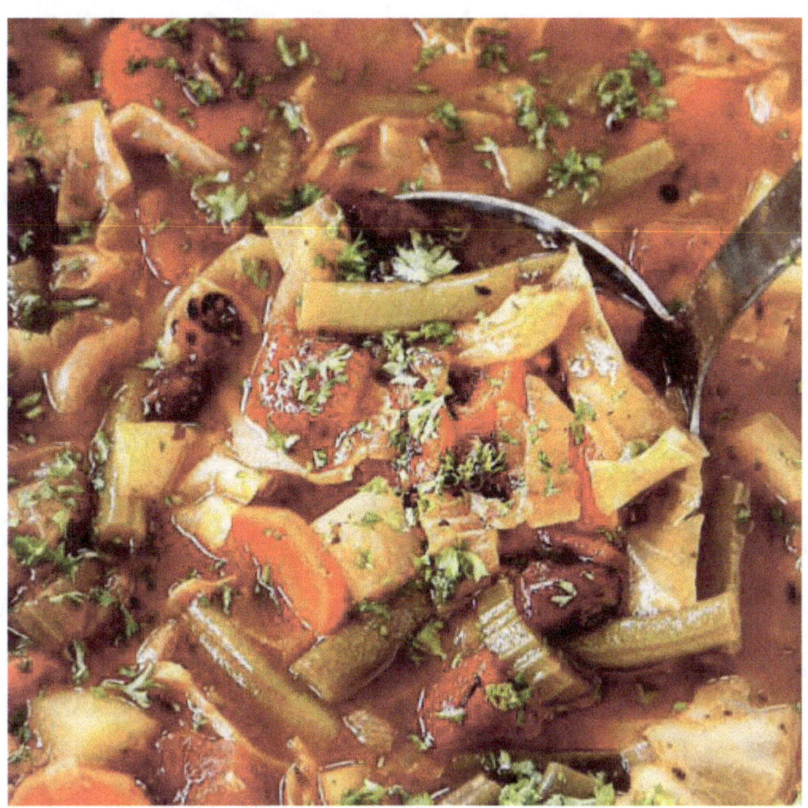

Ingredients:

- 1 head cabbage, shredded

- 1 onion, diced

- 2 carrots, sliced

- 2 celery stalks, chopped

- 4 cups vegetable broth

- 1 can (14 oz) diced tomatoes

- 1 tsp dried oregano - 1 tsp paprika

- Salt and pepper to taste

Tips:

Incorporate a mix of colorful vegetables for diverse nutrients.

Adjust seasoning to personal preference.

Make a large batch for easy meal prep.

Nutritional Information (per serving):

Calories: 120

Protein: 4g

Carbohydrates: 18g

Fat: 4g

Fiber: 6g

Instructions:

1. In a large pot, combine cabbage, onion, carrots, celery, vegetable broth, diced tomatoes, oregano, and paprika.

2. Bring to a boil, then simmer until vegetables are tender.

3. Season with salt and pepper to taste.

8. Prosciutto-wrapped Haddock with Celeriac Mash

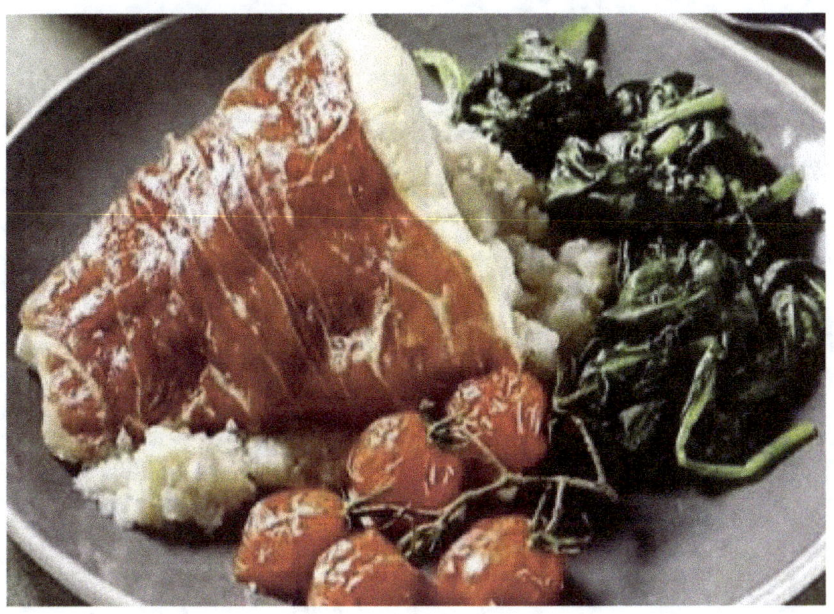

Ingredients:

- 4 haddock fillets

- 8 slices prosciutto

- 2 tbsp olive oil

- 1 celeriac, peeled and diced

- 2 tbsp butter

- 1/2 cup milk

- Salt and pepper to taste

Instructions:

1. Wrap each haddock fillet with 2 slices of prosciutto.

2. Heat olive oil in a pan and cook the haddock until prosciutto is crispy.

3. Boil celeriac until tender, then mash with butter and milk.

4. Season celeriac mash with salt and pepper.

5. Serve prosciutto-wrapped haddock on a bed of celeriac mash.

Tips:

Choose sustainably sourced haddock for an eco-friendly option.

Grill or bake instead of frying for a lighter preparation.

Experiment with herbs like thyme or dill for added flavor.

Nutritional Information (per serving):

Calories: 320

Protein: 28g

Carbohydrates: 10g

Fat: 18g

Fiber: 2g

9. Tofu Pho

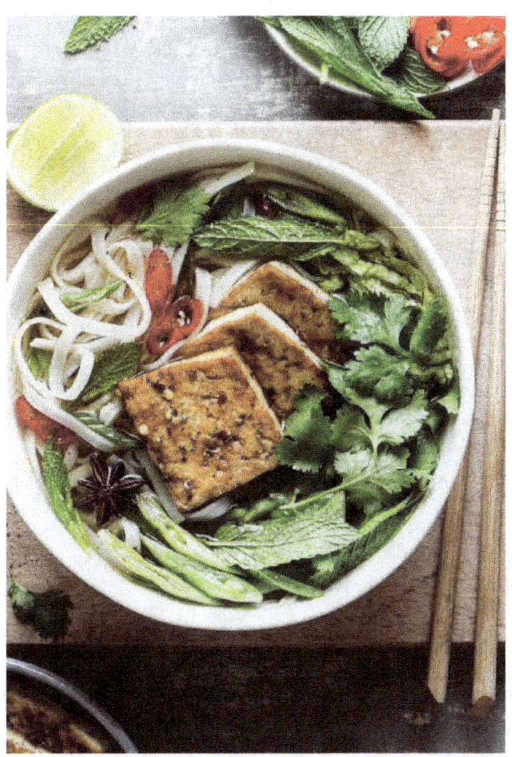

Ingredients:

- 8 cups vegetable broth

- 1 package rice noodles

- 1 block firm tofu, cubed

- 1 cup bean sprouts

- 1 lime, sliced

- Fresh basil and mint leaves

- Sriracha and hoisin sauce for serving

Instructions:

1. Bring vegetable broth to a simmer.

2. Cook rice noodles according to package instructions.

3. Divide noodles among bowls, add tofu, bean sprouts, lime slices, basil, and mint.

4. Pour hot broth over ingredients in each bowl.

5. Serve with Sriracha and hoisin sauce on the side.

Tips:

Select firm tofu for better texture in the soup.

Customize with additional vegetables like bok choy or mushrooms.

Control sodium by using low-sodium vegetable broth.

Nutritional Information (per serving):

Calories: 280

Protein: 16g

Carbohydrates: 35g

Fat: 10g

Fiber: 4g

10. Roasted Vegetable Tacos with Slaw

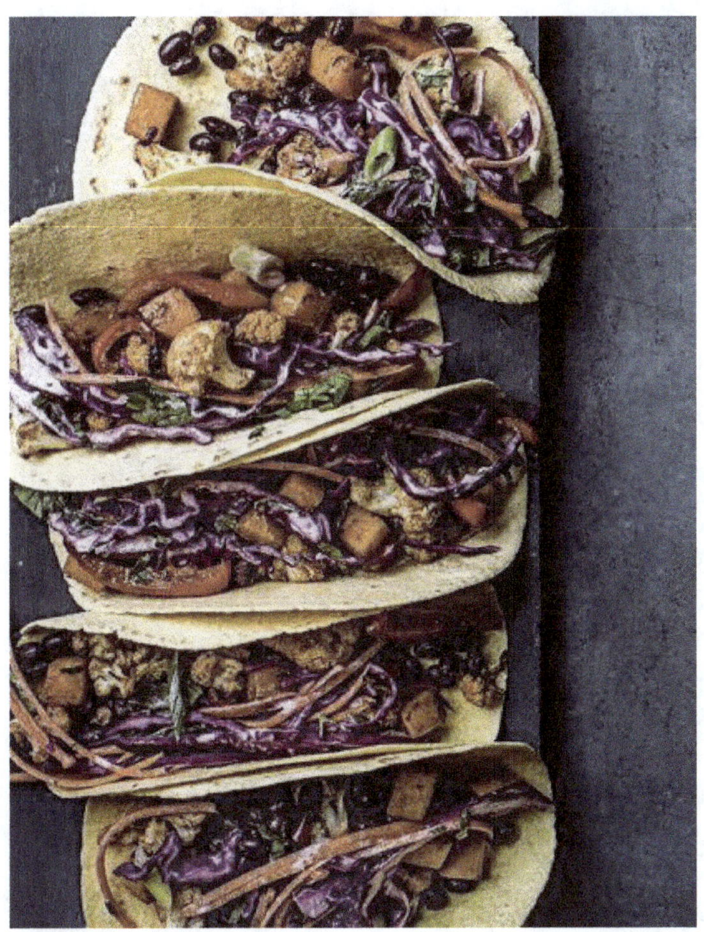

Ingredients:

- 2 bell peppers, sliced - 1 zucchini, sliced

- 1 red onion, sliced - 2 tbsp olive oil

- 1 tsp cumin - 1 tsp chili powder

- Corn tortillas - Cabbage slaw

 - Avocado slices

Instructions:

1. Toss bell peppers, zucchini, and red onion with olive oil, cumin, and chili powder.

2. Roast in the oven until vegetables are tender.

3. Fill corn tortillas with roasted vegetables.

4. Top with cabbage slaw and avocado slices.

Tips:

Use a variety of colorful vegetables for a nutrient-rich filling.

Choose whole-grain corn tortillas for added fiber.

Top with Greek yogurt instead of sour cream for a healthier option.

Nutritional Information (per serving):

Calories: 240

Protein: 8g

Carbohydrates: 30g

Fat: 10g

Fiber: 6g

11. Gluten-free Beef Lasagne

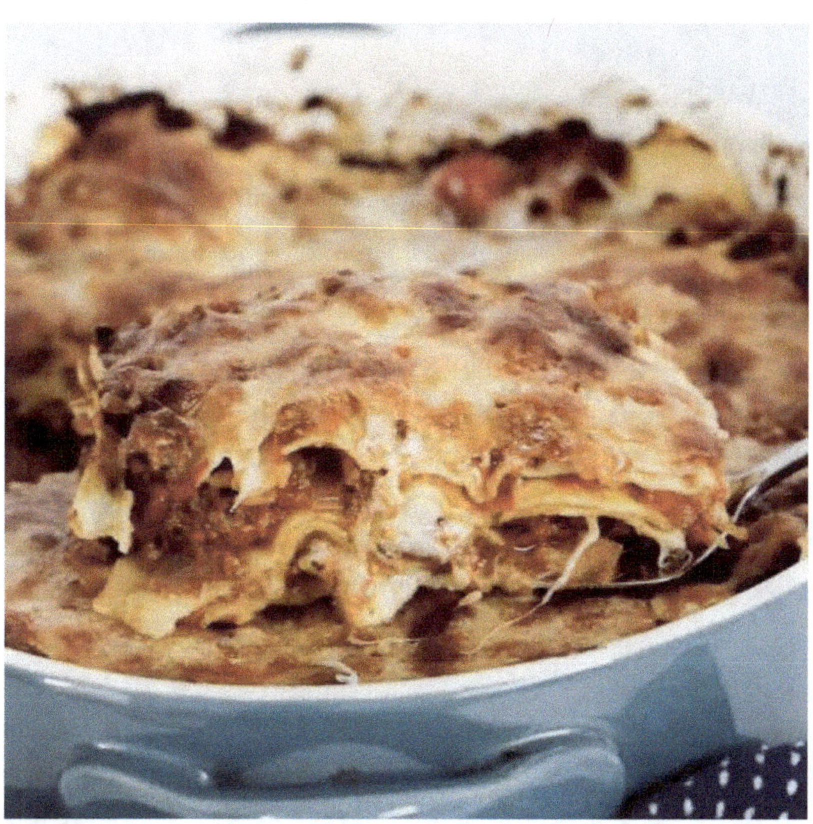

Ingredients:

- 1 lb ground beef - 1 onion, diced

- 2 cloves garlic, minced

- 1 can (14 oz) crushed tomatoes

- 2 cups tomato sauce - 1 tsp dried oregano

- Gluten-free lasagna noodles - 2 cups ricotta cheese

- 2 cups shredded mozzarella

Instructions:

1. Brown ground beef with onion and garlic.

2. Add crushed tomatoes, tomato sauce, and oregano. Simmer.

3. Layer gluten-free lasagna noodles, meat sauce, ricotta, and mozzarella in a baking dish.

4. Repeat layers, finishing with cheese on top.

5. Bake until bubbly and golden.

Tips:

Opt for lean ground beef or turkey to reduce saturated fat.

Experiment with gluten-free lasagna noodles or zucchini slices.

Include spinach or kale layers for added nutrients.

Nutritional Information (per serving):

Calories: 380

Protein: 22g

Carbohydrates: 30g

Fat: 20g

Fiber: 4g

12. Meatball, Tomato & Mozzarella Traybake

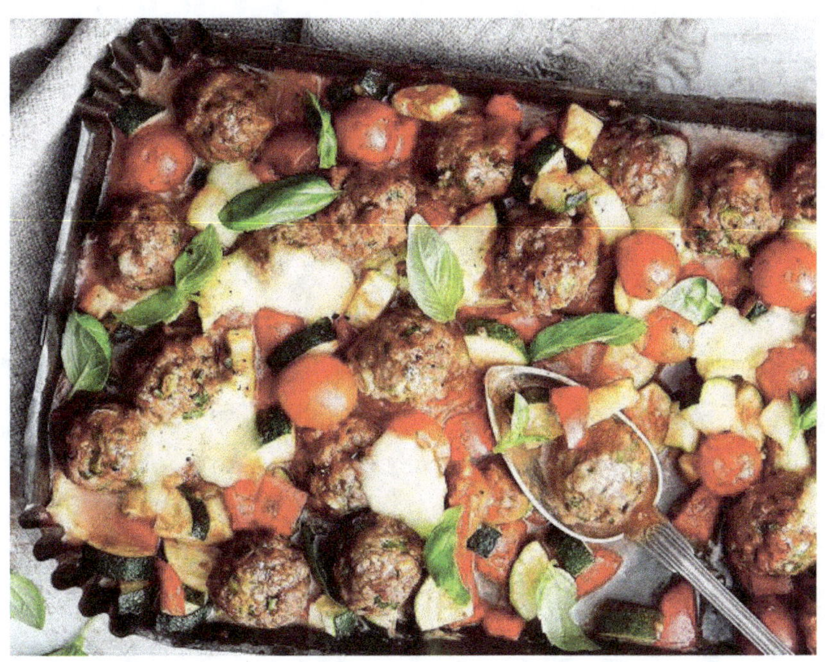

Ingredients:

- 1 lb ground pork

- 1/2 cup breadcrumbs

- 1 egg

- 1 tsp Italian seasoning

- 1 can (14 oz) cherry tomatoes

- 1 cup mozzarella, shredded

- Fresh basil leaves

Instructions:

1. Combine ground pork, breadcrumbs, egg, and Italian seasoning. Form meatballs.

2. Arrange meatballs in a baking dish, add cherry tomatoes.

3. Bake until meatballs are cooked through.

4. Sprinkle with shredded mozzarella and broil until melted.

5. Garnish with fresh basil leaves before serving.

Tips:

Make homemade meatballs with lean ground meat.

Choose part-skim mozzarella for a lighter cheese option.

Add a variety of colorful bell peppers for extra vitamins.

Nutritional Information (per serving):

Calories: 280

Protein: 20g

Carbohydrates: 15g

Fat: 16g

Fiber: 2g

<h1 style="text-align:center">13. Plum Crumble Tart</h1>

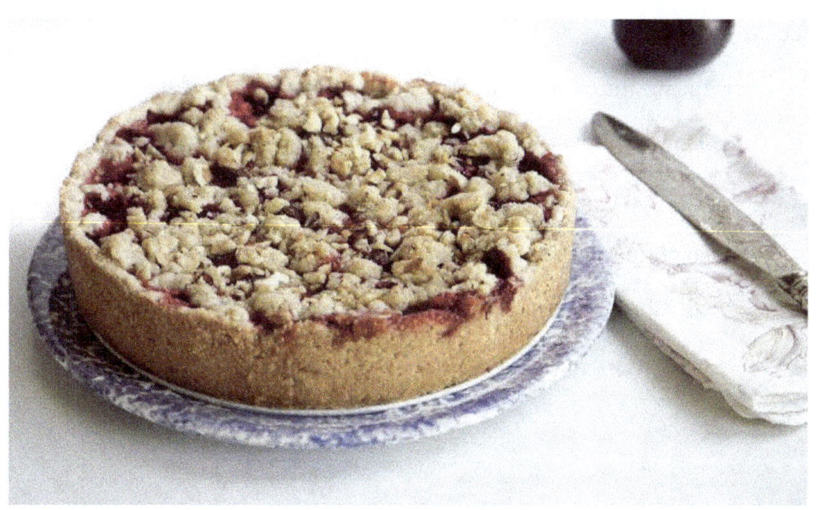

Ingredients:

- 1 1/2 cups all-purpose flour

- 1/2 cup almond flour

- 1/2 cup cold butter, cubed - 1/4 cup sugar

- 4 cups plums, pitted and sliced

- 1/2 cup sugar (for plums)

- 1 tbsp cornstarch

- 1 tsp vanilla extract - 1/2 cup rolled oats

Instructions:

1. Preheat oven to 375°F (190°C).

2. In a bowl, combine all-purpose flour, almond flour, cold butter, and sugar until crumbly.

3. Press the mixture into a tart pan to form the crust.

4. In a separate bowl, toss plums with sugar, cornstarch, and vanilla extract.

5. Arrange plum mixture over the crust.

6. Sprinkle rolled oats on top.

7. Bake for 35-40 minutes or until the crust is golden and plums are bubbly.

Tips:

Select ripe plums for sweetness and flavor.

Experiment with a mix of whole-grain and almond flour for a nutty crust.

Serve with a dollop of Greek yogurt for added protein.

Nutritional Information (per serving):

Calories: 280

Protein: 5g

Carbohydrates: 40g

Fat: 12g

Fiber: 4g

14. Butternut Squash Galette

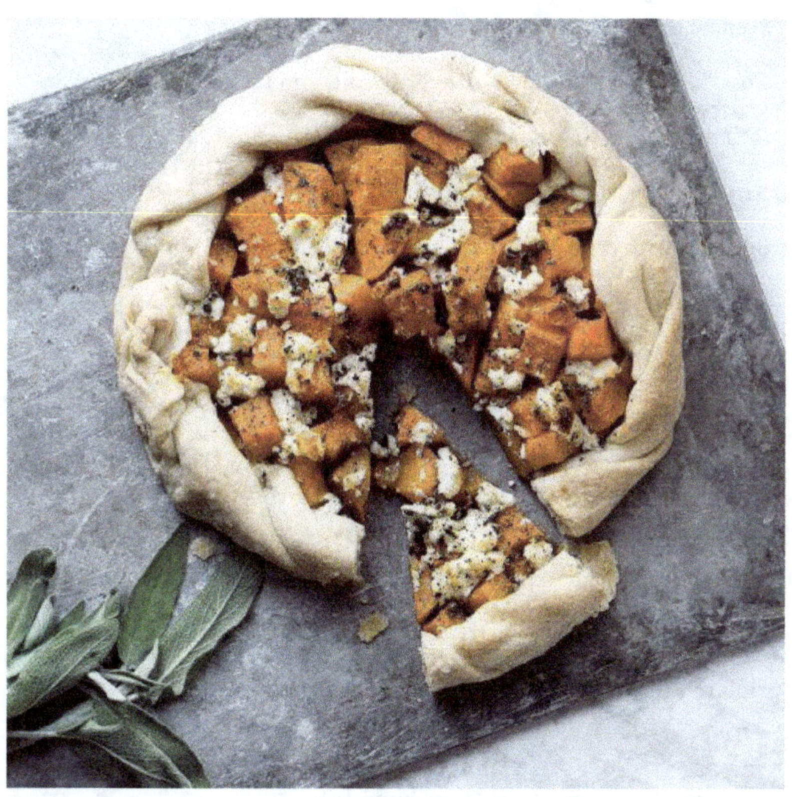

Ingredients:

- 1 1/2 cups butternut squash, peeled and thinly sliced

- 1 tbsp olive oil - Salt and pepper to taste

- 1 sheet puff pastry, thawed - 1/2 cup goat cheese, crumbled

- 1/4 cup walnuts, chopped - 1 tbsp honey

Instructions:

1. Preheat oven to 400°F (200°C).

2. Toss butternut squash with olive oil, salt, and pepper.

3. Roll out puff pastry on a baking sheet.

4. Arrange butternut squash slices in the center.

5. Sprinkle with crumbled goat cheese and chopped walnuts.

6. Fold the edges of the pastry over the filling.

7. Bake for 25-30 minutes or until golden. Drizzle with honey before serving.

Tips:

Use pre-cut butternut squash for a time-saving option.

Choose whole-grain puff pastry for added fiber.

Sprinkle with pumpkin seeds for extra crunch and nutrition.

Nutritional Information (per serving):

Calories: 320

Protein: 6g

Carbohydrates: 30g

Fat: 20g

Fiber: 4g

DINNER

15. Teriyaki Chicken Sheet Pan

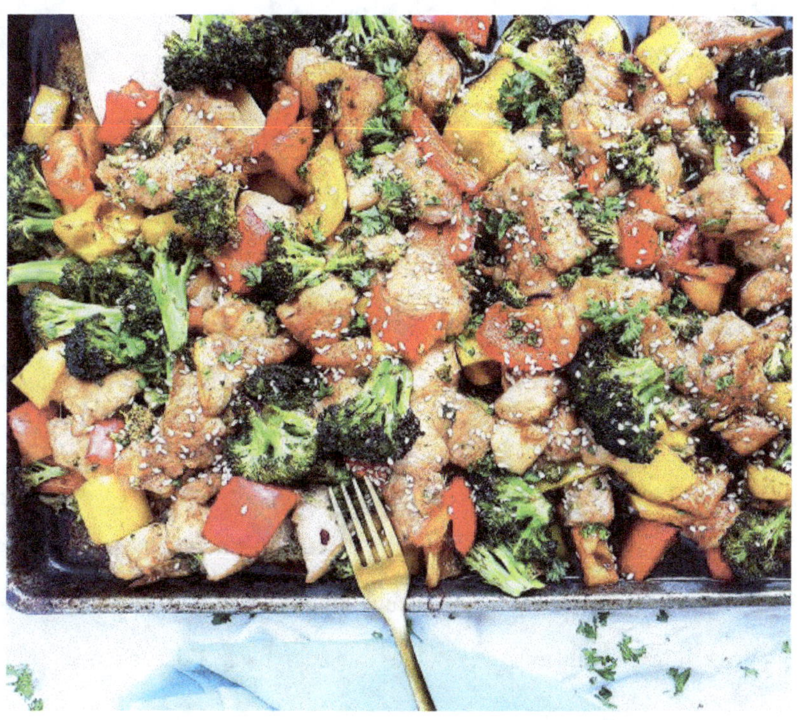

Ingredients:

- 1 lb (450g) chicken breast, thinly sliced

- 2 cups broccoli florets

- 1 cup bell peppers, sliced

- 1 cup carrots, julienned

- 1/2 cup teriyaki sauce - 2 tablespoons olive oil

- Salt and pepper to taste

Instructions:

1. Preheat oven to 400°F (200°C).

2. Place sliced chicken, broccoli, bell peppers, and carrots on a sheet pan.

3. Drizzle with 2 tablespoons of olive oil and teriyaki sauce.

4. Season with salt and pepper.

5. Toss everything to coat evenly.

6. Roast in the oven for 20-25 minutes or until chicken is cooked through.

Tips:

Use low-sodium teriyaki sauce to reduce sodium intake.

Experiment with additional vegetables like snap peas or asparagus.

Nutritional Information (per serving):

Calories: ~350

Protein: ~30g

Carbohydrates: ~20g

Fat: ~15g

<h1 align="center">16. Vegetarian Black Bean Chili</h1>

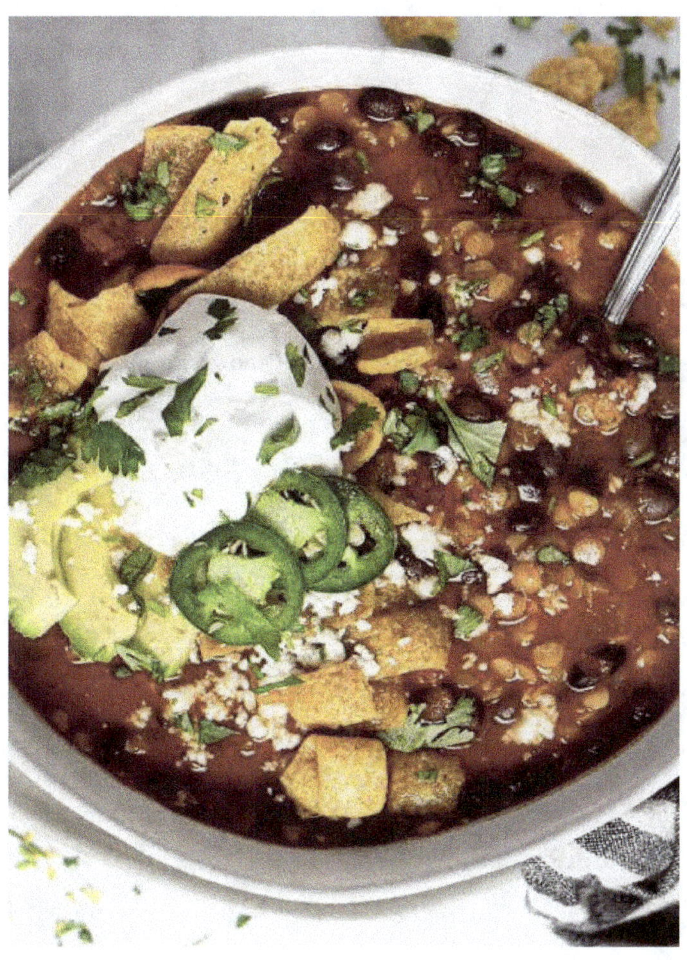

Ingredients:

- 2 cans (15 oz each) black beans, drained and rinsed

- 1 onion, diced - 2 bell peppers, diced

- 3 cloves garlic, minced

- 1 can (28 oz) crushed tomatoes

- 2 tablespoons chili powder

- 1 tablespoon cumin

- Salt and pepper to taste

Instructions:

1. In a large pot, sauté onions, bell peppers, and garlic until softened.

2. Add black beans, crushed tomatoes, chili powder, cumin, salt, and pepper.

3. Simmer for 20-25 minutes, stirring occasionally.

Tips:

Add a variety of beans for texture and nutritional diversity.

Top with Greek yogurt and cilantro for added flavor.

Nutritional Information (per serving):

Calories: ~300

Protein: ~15g

Carbohydrates: ~45g

Fat: ~5g

17. Mushroom Stroganoff

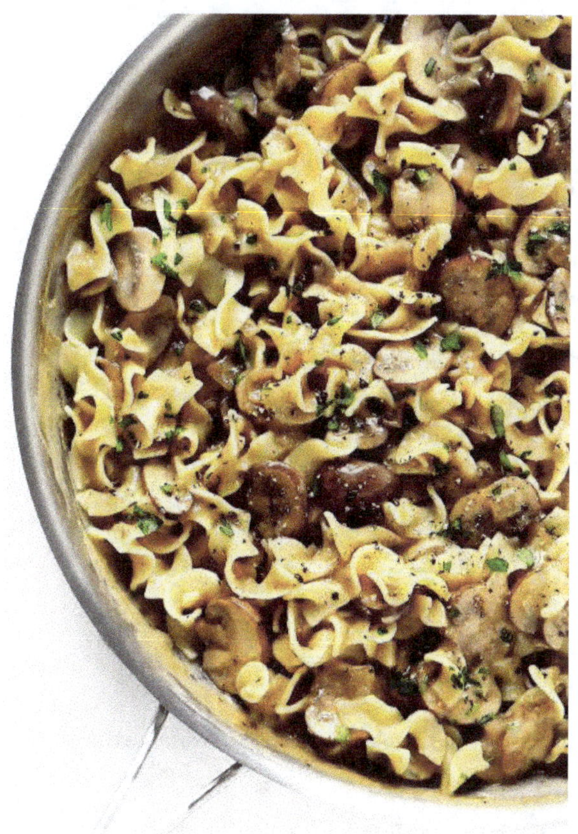

Ingredients:

- 1 lb (450g) mushrooms, sliced

- 1 onion, finely chopped

- 2 cloves garlic, minced

- 1 cup vegetable broth

- 1 cup Greek yogurt - 2 tablespoons flour

- 2 tablespoons olive oil

- Salt and pepper to taste

Instructions:

1. In a pan, sauté mushrooms, onions, and garlic in olive oil until mushrooms are golden.

2. Sprinkle flour over the mixture and stir.

3. Gradually add vegetable broth, stirring continuously.

4. Simmer for 10 minutes, then stir in Greek yogurt.

5. Season with salt and pepper.

Tips:

Choose whole-grain pasta for added fiber.

Consider using low-fat Greek yogurt for a creamy texture.

Nutritional Information (per serving):

Calories: ~250

Protein: ~10g

Carbohydrates: ~30g

Fat: ~10g

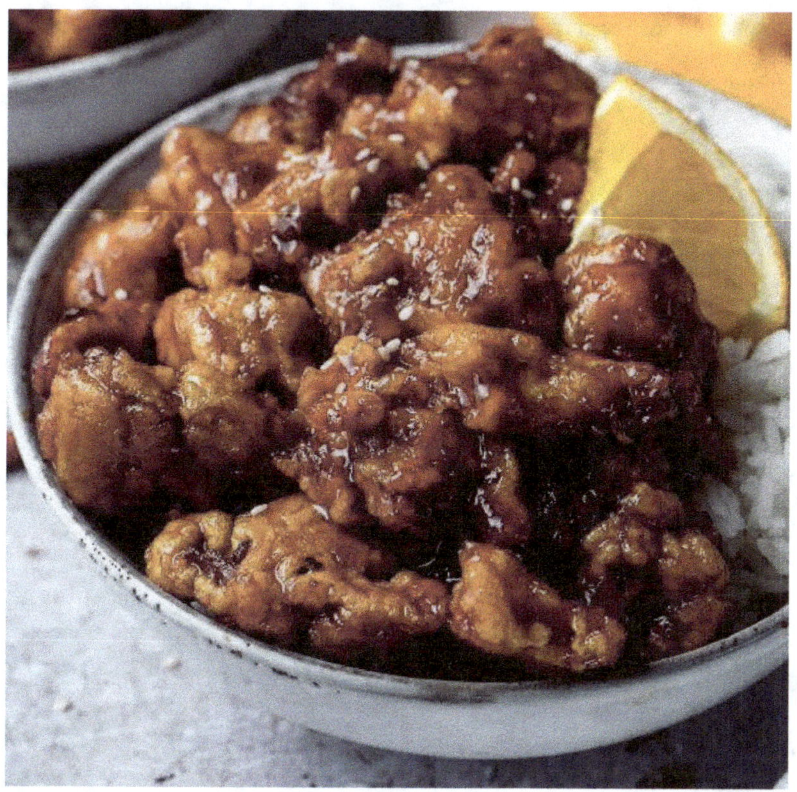

Ingredients:

- 1 lb (450g) boneless, skinless chicken thighs, diced

- 1/2 cup orange juice

- 2 tablespoons soy sauce

- 2 tablespoons honey - 1 tablespoon cornstarch

- 1 tablespoon sesame oil - 2 cloves garlic, minced

- 1 teaspoon ginger, grated

- Green onions for garnish

- Sesame seeds for garnish

Instructions:

1. In a bowl, mix orange juice, soy sauce, honey, and cornstarch to create the sauce.

2. Heat sesame oil in a pan, add garlic and ginger, sauté until fragrant.

3. Add diced chicken, cook until browned.

4. Pour in the orange sauce, simmer until the sauce thickens.

5. Garnish with green onions and sesame seeds.

Tips:

Opt for skinless chicken for a leaner dish.

Serve over cauliflower rice for a lower-carb option.

Nutritional Information (per serving):

Calories: ~400

Protein: ~25g

Carbohydrates: ~35g

Fat: ~15g

19. Chicken Cacciatore

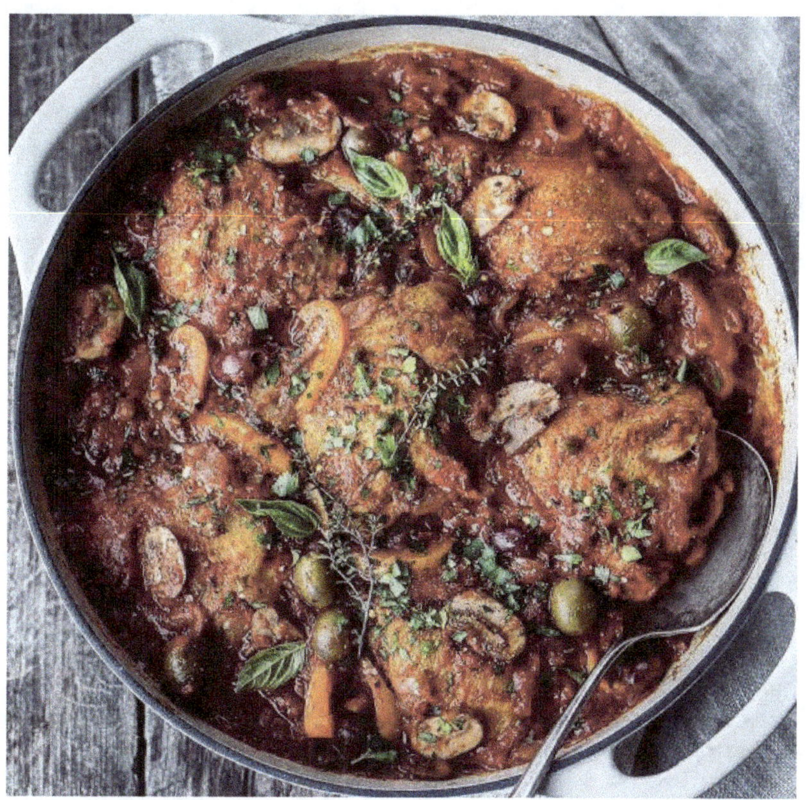

Ingredients:

- 1 lb (450g) chicken thighs, bone-in

- 1 can (14 oz) diced tomatoes

- 1 onion, diced - 1 bell pepper, sliced

- 2 cloves garlic, minced

- 1/2 cup red wine

- 2 tablespoons olive oil

- 1 teaspoon dried oregano

- 1 teaspoon dried basil

- Salt and pepper to taste

Instructions:

1. Season chicken thighs with salt, pepper, oregano, and basil.

2. Heat olive oil in a skillet, brown chicken on both sides.

3. Add diced tomatoes, onion, bell pepper, and garlic.

4. Pour in red wine, bring to a simmer, cover, and cook for 25-30 minutes.

Tips:

Choose skinless chicken to reduce saturated fat.

Add extra vegetables such as zucchini or bell peppers.

Nutritional Information (per serving):

Calories: ~300

Protein: ~20g

Carbohydrates: ~20g

Fat: ~15g

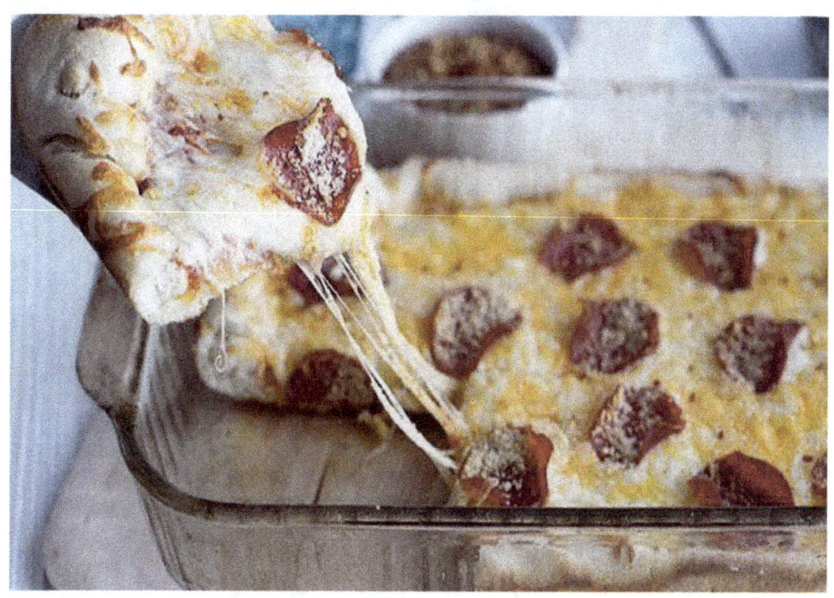

20. Deep Dish Pizza Casserole

Ingredients:

- 2 cups whole wheat penne pasta

- 1 lb (450g) lean ground turkey

- 1 cup bell peppers, diced

- 1 cup mushrooms, sliced

- 1 can (14 oz) crushed tomatoes

- 1 teaspoon dried oregano

- 1 teaspoon dried basil

- 1/2 cup part-skim mozzarella, shredded

- 1/4 cup Parmesan cheese, grated

Instructions:

1. Cook pasta according to package instructions, drain, and set aside.

2. In a skillet, brown ground turkey.

3. Add bell peppers, mushrooms, crushed tomatoes, oregano, and basil.

4. Simmer for 10-15 minutes.

5. In a baking dish, layer cooked pasta, turkey mixture, and top with cheeses.

6. Bake at 375°F (190°C) for 20-25 minutes or until cheese is melted and bubbly.

Tips:

Choose lean ground turkey for a healthier option.

Load up on additional veggies like spinach or mushrooms.

Nutritional Information (per serving):

Calories: ~350

Protein: ~25g

Carbohydrates: ~40g

Fat: ~10g

21. Honey Garlic Pork Chops

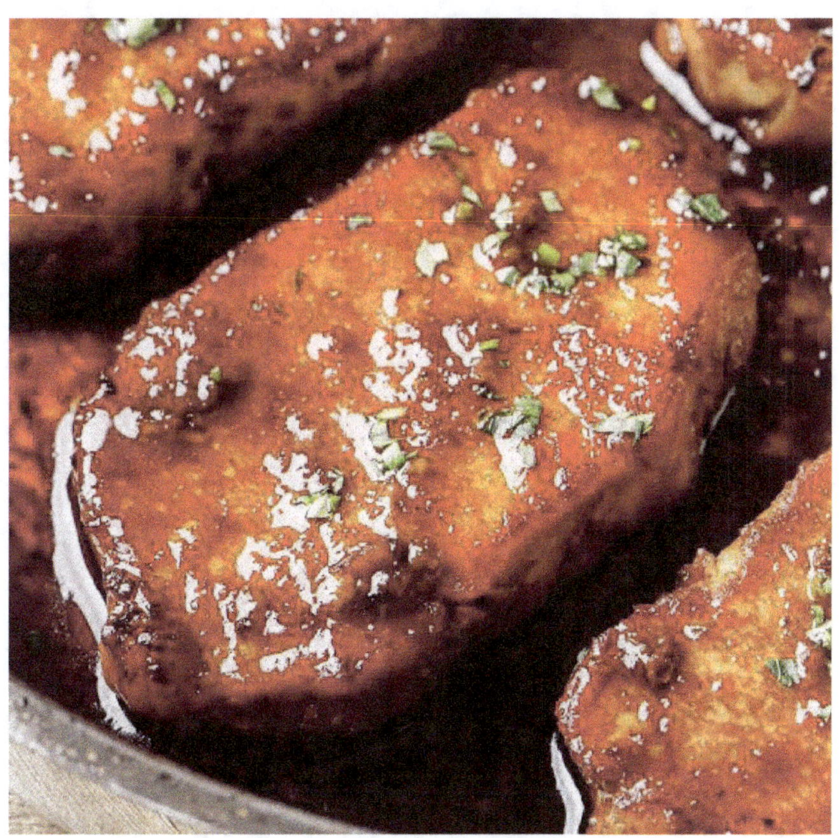

Ingredients:

- 4 boneless pork chops

- 1/4 cup honey

- 3 tablespoons soy sauce

- 2 cloves garlic, minced

- 1 teaspoon ginger, grated

- 1 tablespoon olive oil

- Salt and pepper to taste

Instructions:

1. Season pork chops with salt and pepper.

2. In a bowl, mix honey, soy sauce, garlic, and ginger.

3. Heat olive oil in a skillet, sear pork chops on both sides.

4. Pour honey-garlic mixture over chops, cook until glazed.

Tips:

Marinate the pork chops for extra flavor.

Grill or bake instead of frying for a lighter version.

Nutritional Information (per serving):

Calories: ~300

Protein: ~30g

Carbohydrates: ~15g

Fat: ~12g

22. Mustard Glazed Salmon with Lentils

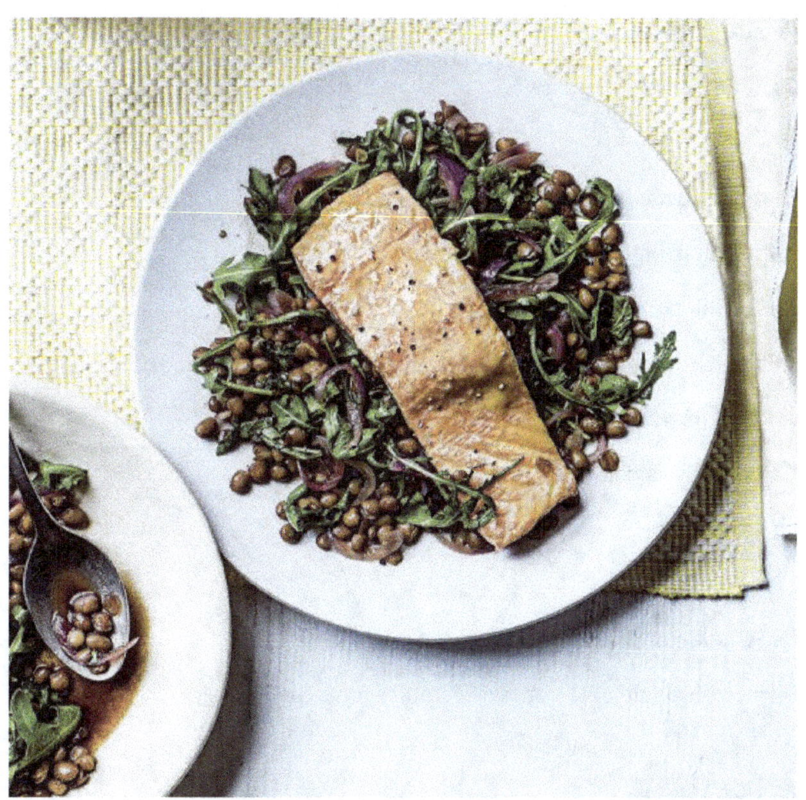

Ingredients:

- 4 salmon fillets

- 1/4 cup Dijon mustard

- 2 tablespoons maple syrup

- 1 tablespoon olive oil

- 1 cup cooked lentils

- 1 cup spinach, chopped

- Salt and pepper to taste

Instructions:

1. Preheat oven to 400°F (200°C).

2. Mix Dijon mustard, maple syrup, and olive oil.

3. Place salmon on a baking sheet, brush with mustard mixture.

4. Roast for 12-15 minutes.

5. Serve over a bed of cooked lentils and spinach.

Tips:

Use whole-grain mustard for added texture.

Serve with a side of steamed vegetables for more fiber.

Nutritional Information (per serving):

Calories: ~400

Protein: ~30g

Carbohydrates: ~30g

Fat: ~18g

23. Boodles with Harissa Meatballs

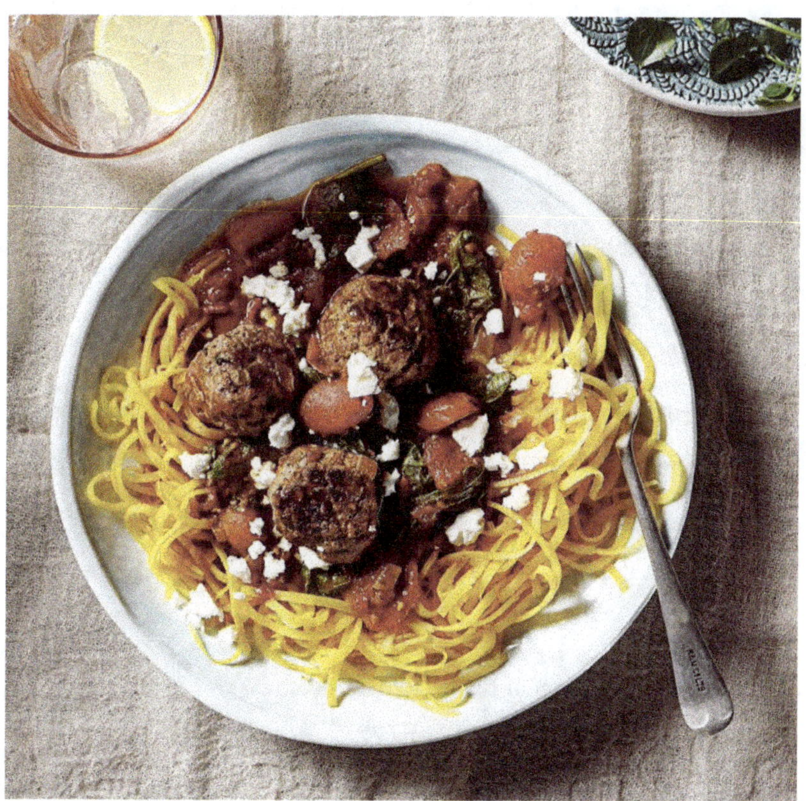

Ingredients:

- 1 lb (450g) lean ground beef

- 2 tablespoons harissa paste

- 1/2 cup breadcrumbs

- 1 egg - 2 zucchinis, spiralized (boodles)

- 1 can (14 oz) diced tomatoes

- 1 onion, diced

- 2 cloves garlic, minced

- 1 tablespoon olive oil - Fresh parsley for garnish

Instructions:

1. In a bowl, combine ground beef, harissa, breadcrumbs, and egg. Form into meatballs.

2. In a skillet, heat olive oil, brown meatballs.

3. Add diced tomatoes, onion, and garlic, simmer until meatballs are cooked through.

4. Serve meatballs over zucchini noodles, garnish with fresh parsley.

Tips:

Opt for lean ground beef or turkey for the meatballs.

Use whole wheat or lentil-based pasta for a nutrient boost.

Nutritional Information (per serving):

Calories: ~350

Protein: ~20g

Carbohydrates: ~40g

Fat: ~12g

24. Sausages with Chickpea Mash & Braised Red Cabbage

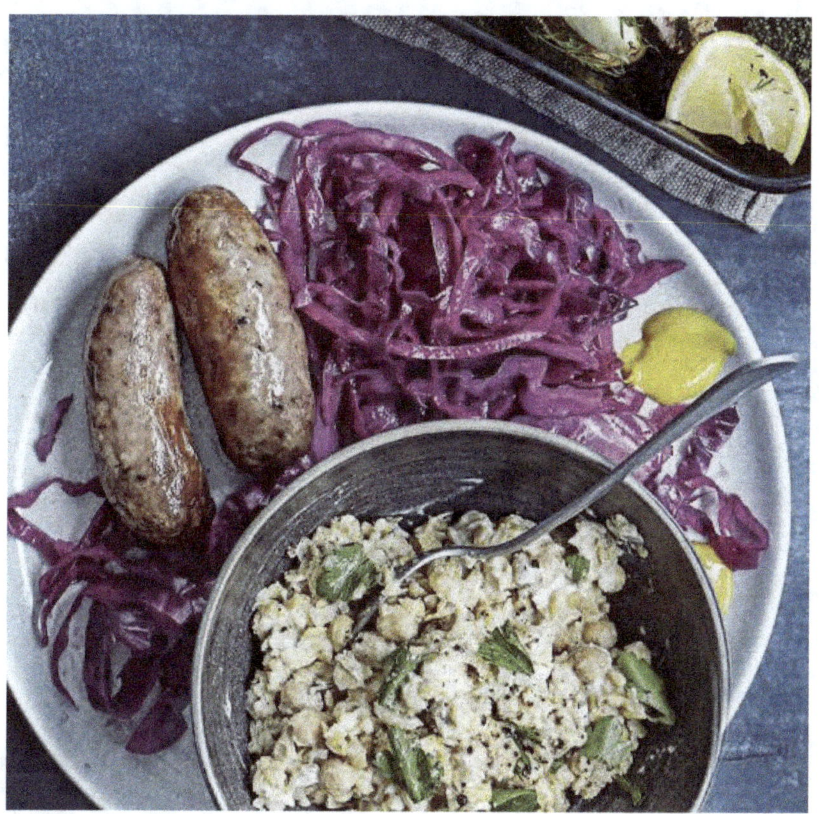

Ingredients:

- 1 lb (450g) chicken or turkey sausages

- 2 cans (15 oz each) chickpeas, drained and rinsed

- 1/2 cup chicken broth

- 1 head red cabbage, shredded

- 2 tablespoons apple cider vinegar

- 1 tablespoon olive oil

- Salt and pepper to taste

Instructions:

1. Grill or cook sausages according to package instructions.

2. In a pan, sauté chickpeas in olive oil, add chicken broth, mash slightly.

3. In a separate pan, braise shredded red cabbage with apple cider vinegar until tender.

4. Serve sausages over chickpea mash with a side of braised red cabbage.

Tips:

Choose lean chicken or turkey sausages.

Increase cabbage for added fiber and vitamins.

Nutritional Information (per serving):

Calories: ~400

Protein: ~20g

Carbohydrates: ~30g

Fat: ~20g

25. Spaghetti Arrabbiata with Squid

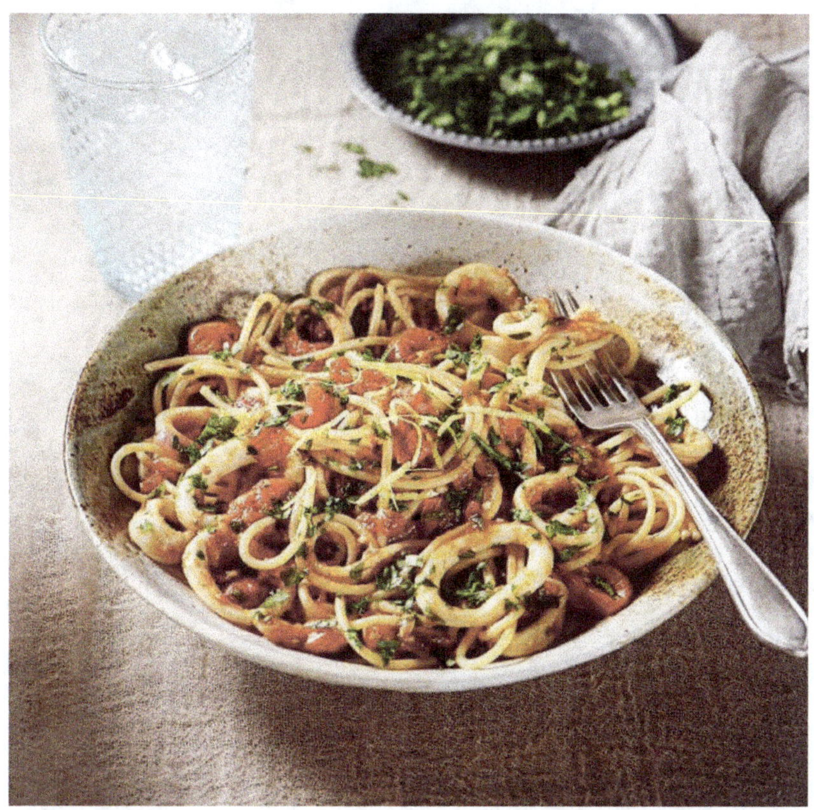

Ingredients:

- 8 oz (225g) whole wheat spaghetti

- 1 lb (450g) squid tubes, cleaned and sliced

- 1 can (14 oz) diced tomatoes

- 3 cloves garlic, minced

- 1 teaspoon red pepper flakes

- 2 tablespoons olive oil

- Fresh basil for garnish

- Salt and pepper to taste

Instructions:

1. Cook spaghetti according to package instructions.

2. In a pan, sauté garlic and red pepper flakes in olive oil.

3. Add sliced squid, cook until opaque.

4. Pour in diced tomatoes, simmer for 10 minutes.

5. Toss cooked spaghetti in the squid and tomato mixture.

6. Garnish with fresh basil.

Tips:

Select whole wheat or alternative grain spaghetti.

Increase veggies like cherry tomatoes or spinach.

Nutritional Information (per serving):

Calories: ~350

Protein: ~25g

Carbohydrates: ~40g

Fat: ~10g

26. Prawn Singapore Noodles

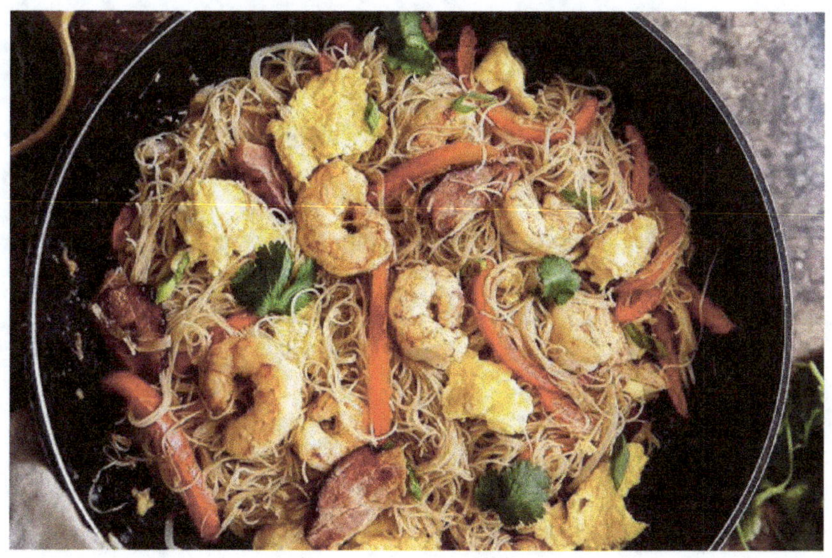

Ingredients:

- 8 oz (225g) rice vermicelli noodles

- 1 lb (450g) large prawns, peeled and deveined

- 1 cup bean sprouts

- 1 bell pepper, julienned

- 1 carrot, julienned

- 2 cloves garlic, minced

- 2 tablespoons curry powder

- 2 tablespoons soy sauce

- 1 tablespoon sesame oil

- Green onions for garnish

Instructions:

1. Cook rice vermicelli according to package instructions, drain, and set aside.

2. In a wok, heat sesame oil, sauté garlic until fragrant.

3. Add prawns, bell pepper, and carrot, stir-fry until prawns are pink.

4. Sprinkle curry powder, add cooked noodles, soy sauce, and bean sprouts. Toss to combine.

5. Garnish with green onions.

Tips:

Use whole grain noodles for added fiber.

Stir-fry quickly to retain the crunchiness of vegetables.

Nutritional Information (per serving):

Calories: ~350

Protein: ~25g

Carbohydrates: ~45g

Fat: ~8g

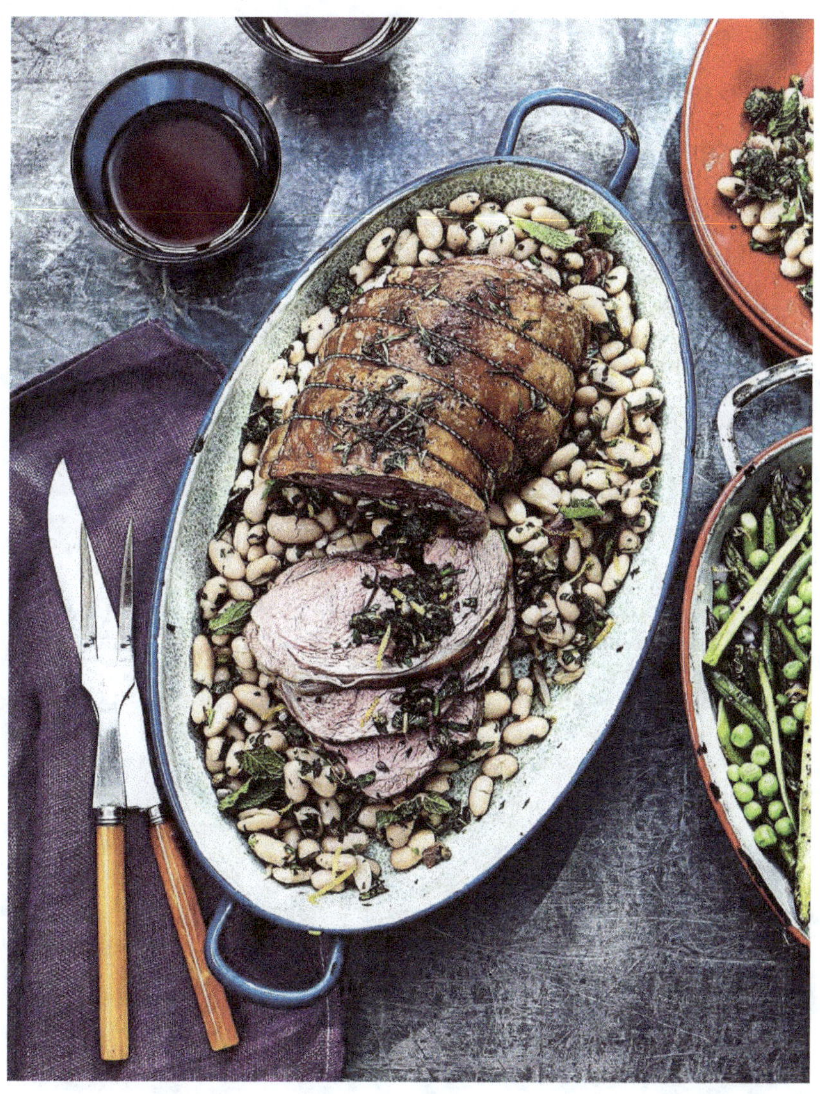

Ingredients:

- 1 lb (450g) lamb leg, boneless

- 2 cans (15 oz each) cannellini beans, drained and rinsed

- 1 cup cherry tomatoes, halved

- 1/2 cup fresh parsley, chopped

- 2 tablespoons capers

- 2 tablespoons olive oil

- 1 lemon, juiced

- Salt and pepper to taste

Instructions:

1. Preheat oven to 375°F (190°C).

2. Rub lamb with olive oil, salt, and pepper. Roast for 25-30 minutes.

3. In a bowl, mix cannellini beans, cherry tomatoes, parsley, capers, olive oil, and lemon juice.

4. Serve roasted lamb over the salsa verde beans.

Tips:

Trim visible fat from the lamb for a leaner dish.

Experiment with different herbs for the salsa verde.

Nutritional Information (per serving):

Calories: ~400

Protein: ~30g

Carbohydrates: ~30g

Fat: ~18g

28. Glazed Gammon with Pineapple & Egg-Fried Rice

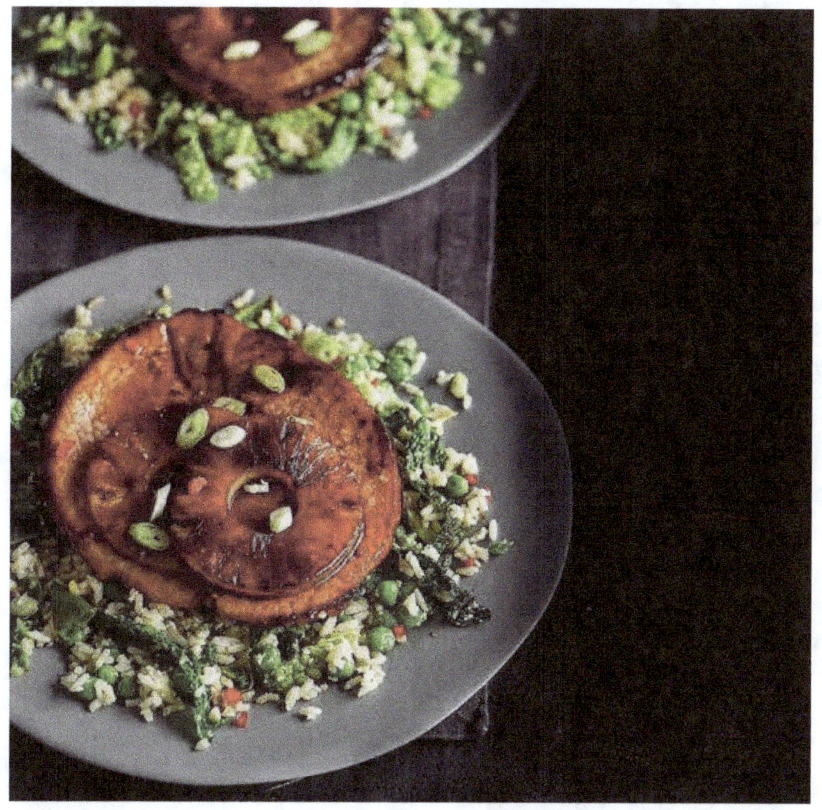

Ingredients:

- 1 lb (450g) gammon steak

- 2 cups cooked brown rice

- 1 cup pineapple, diced

- 2 eggs, beaten

- 1 cup frozen peas

- 2 tablespoons soy sauce

- 1 tablespoon honey

- 1 tablespoon vegetable oil

- Green onions for garnish

Instructions:

1. Grill or cook gammon steak according to package instructions.

2. In a wok, heat vegetable oil, add beaten eggs, scramble.

3. Add cooked rice, pineapple, and frozen peas. Stir-fry for 5 minutes.

4. In a small bowl, mix soy sauce and honey. Pour over the rice mixture.

5. Slice gammon and serve over pineapple and egg-fried rice. Garnish with green onions.

Tips:

Choose lean cuts of gammon for lower fat content.

Use brown rice for a higher fiber option.

Nutritional Information (per serving):

Calories: ~350

Protein: ~25g

Carbohydrates: ~40g

Fat: ~10g

29. Honey & Soy Glazed Ham

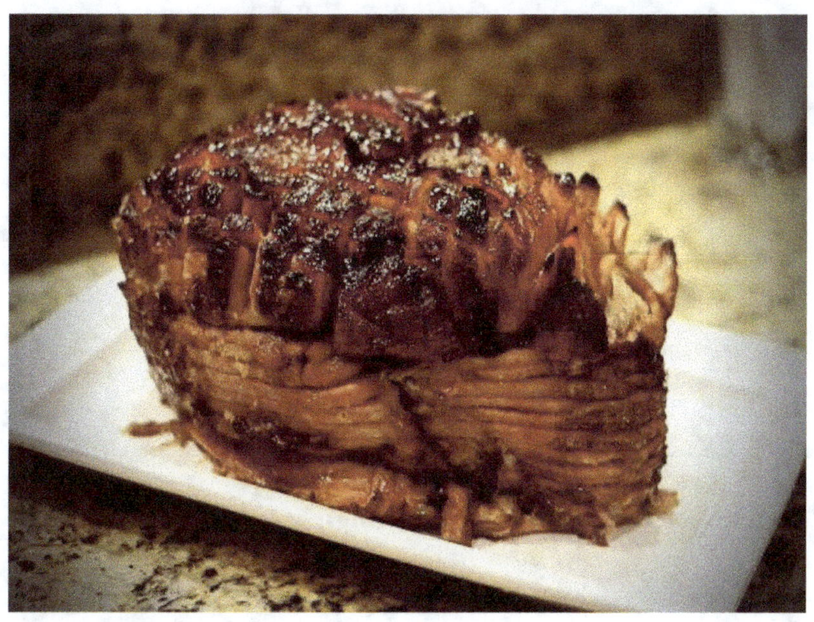

Ingredients:

- 1 lb (450g) ham, fully cooked

- 1/2 cup honey - 3 tablespoons soy sauce

- 2 tablespoons Dijon mustard

- 1 tablespoon olive oil

- 1 teaspoon garlic powder

- 1/2 teaspoon ground ginger

Instructions:

1. Preheat the oven to 350°F (175°C).

2. In a bowl, whisk together honey, soy sauce, Dijon mustard, olive oil, garlic powder, and ground ginger.

3. Place ham in a roasting pan, brush with the honey-soy glaze.

4. Roast for 20-25 minutes, basting with the glaze every 10 minutes.

Tips:

Opt for a leaner cut of ham to reduce fat content.

Use low-sodium soy sauce to control sodium intake.

Nutritional Information (per serving):

Calories: ~300

Protein: ~25g

Carbohydrates: ~10g

Fat: ~15g

KITCHEN NECESSARY TOOLS

Note that these detailed explanations should provide a clearer understanding of each kitchen instrument's purpose and how to effectively use them for the specified recipes.

1. Sheet Pan:

- Function: A large, flat pan with raised edges used for baking and roasting. It allows for even cooking of various ingredients.

- How to Use: Arrange thinly sliced chicken, broccoli, bell peppers, and carrots on the sheet pan. Drizzle with olive oil and teriyaki sauce, then roast in a preheated oven until the chicken is cooked through.

2. Large Pot:

- Function: Ideal for cooking large quantities of chili, pasta, and stews. It evenly distributes heat, allowing for thorough cooking.

- How to Use: Sauté onions, bell peppers, and garlic in the pot. Add black beans, crushed tomatoes, chili powder, cumin, salt, and pepper. Simmer, stirring occasionally, until the flavors meld.

3. Skillet or Pan:

- Function: Versatile for sautéing, frying, and searing. Provides a wide surface area for cooking ingredients quickly.

- How to Use: Brown chicken in a skillet, add garlic and ginger. Pour in the orange sauce, and simmer until the chicken is glazed and fully cooked.

4. Baking Dish:

- Function: Used for baking casseroles and layered dishes, ensuring even cooking.

- How to Use: Layer cooked pasta, turkey mixture, and cheeses in the baking dish. Bake until the cheese is melted and bubbly.

5. Wok:

- Function: A versatile pan for stir-frying and quick cooking at high temperatures.

- How to Use: Stir-fry prawns, bell pepper, carrot, and noodles quickly in a wok. Tossing ingredients together over high heat ensures a flavorful, well-cooked dish.

6. Grill or Panini Press:

- Function: Ideal for grilling meats, providing a smoky flavor and grill marks.

- How to Use: Grill or cook gammon steak according to package instructions, ensuring it's fully cooked and has grill marks for added flavor.

7. Bowl:

- Function: Essential for mixing and combining ingredients for marinades or sauces.

- How to Use: Whisk together honey, soy sauce, garlic, and ginger in a bowl. Pour the mixture over pork chops for marinating.

8. Oven:

- Function: Used for baking and roasting, providing consistent heat for even cooking.

- How to Use: Preheat the oven for recipes like the mustard-glazed salmon. Roast until the salmon is cooked through.

9. Roasting Pan:

- Function: Specifically designed for roasting larger cuts of meat, such as lamb.

- How to Use: Roast lamb on the rack in the preheated oven until it reaches the desired level of doneness.

10. Wok or Skillet (for Singapore Noodles):

- Function: Essential for stir-frying noodles and vegetables quickly.

- How to Use: Stir-fry prawns, bell pepper, carrot, and noodles quickly in a wok. Tossing ingredients together over high heat ensures a flavorful, well-cooked dish.

11. Blender or Food Processor (for Salsa Verde):

- Function: Used for blending herbs and ingredients into a smooth sauce.

- How to Use: Combine fresh parsley, capers, olive oil, and lemon juice in a blender. Blend until smooth to create a vibrant salsa verde for roasted lamb.